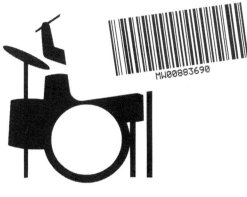

HEALTHY HUSTLE

BECAUSE TOIL ISN'T A SUSTAINABLE LIFE PLAN

ANDREW EDWIN JENKINS

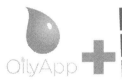

OilyApp +

A BOOK YOU'LL ACTUALLY READ ABOUT TEN OILS FOR LIFE BALANCE

ISBN number – 9781796691139

Connect online!

Podcast-
OilyApp.com

Social-
www.Facebook.com/OilyApp
www.Facebook.com/OilyApp
www.Instagram.com/OilyApp

YouTube-
www.YouTube.com/Overflow

Website-
OilyApp.com
Jenkins.tv

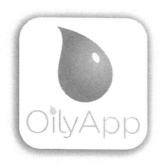

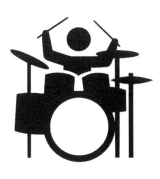

CONTENTS

AN OVERVIEW OF WHERE WE'RE HEADED!

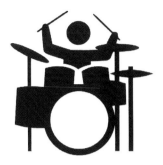

ABOUT THE SERIES
+ ABOUT HUSTLE

We created OilyApp (go to OilyApp.com to learn more) with the goal of educating you about Young Living's vast array of incredible products. The app is uniquely the *only* third party app that's an approved partner of Young Living Essential Oils, passing a strict compliance review each time we update.

OilyApp works well with Young Living's stated mission of taking oils into every home in the world. Once people have the oils, they need to know... *how do we use them?!*

Whereas shipping a desk reference to everyone is cumbersome and difficult (besides, who wants to always lug it around!?), most people have a smart phone. An app is the perfect solution.

Furthermore, the app was created by actual members (Ernie Yarbrough, one of the founders, has his wife are Royal Crown Diamonds). In other words, it was created in the field for use in the field.

THE NEXT THING

After a few years of providing users with OilyApp, it became apparent than another addition was needed for product users and business builders who wanted to go to the "next level." Enter OilyApp+, a web-based experience designed to provide users with more relevant information- things like scripts they could use to learn and/or educate their teams, graphics that were relevant and educational, and access to Diamond+ leaders.

We created OilyApp+ in less than two weeks from its conception.

From the beginning, we knew we wanted the OA+ to include video courses and online scripts- tools you could use to review and then teach your "people" what you were learning.

After a few weeks, the thought hit us: *What if we made the scripts into small books, too- small pocket-sized books people could easily review and use to study, to lead others, and even to teach classes?*

Hence the title you have in your hand.

The script and the videos where we teach the material are available in OA+ (access it all at OilyApp.com).

ABOUT HEALTHY HUSTLE

It seems like Everybody uses the word *hustle* nowadays, tossing it out like candy on Halloween or cheap beads at Mardi Gras.

But what does it REALLY mean? And how can we ACTUALLY DO IT? And, is there a way to do it and sustain everything else we've got going on in life…?.

Maybe, maybe not. Depends on how you define *hustle*.

And it really depends on WHY you're hustling. If you're not careful, it can turn into toil or noise or something worse.

Take the drums in the pic as an example. No musician hustles on stage more than the drummer. They keep the rhythm, they physically push the limits, and they create MUSIC…

But the music happens because of the moments of rest. No rest = all noise.

Rhythm only happens because of the beat of times ON and cadence of times OFF.

Maybe we can learn a lot from the drummer. Maybe we can learn about this thing called hustle and bring some balance in…

In this "short book you'll actually read" we discuss the rhythm of creation (yeah, there really is one), we talk about the wrong reasons we toil, and we determine what healthy hustle looks like. And, in the end, we'll outline ten of the best oils to use for optimal life balance.

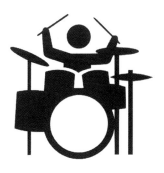

1. CREATION'S RHYTHM

MAIN IDEA= IN MUSIC, THE RESTS ARE AS IMPORTANT AS THE NOTES YOU PLAY. LIFE IS THE SAME WAY. THERE'S A DEFINITE BEAT TO CREATION THAT WORKS WELL FOR US WHEN WE EMBRACE IT.

Over the past few months it hit me: *rest is part of the rhythm of life*. In fact, we're created for rest as much as we're created for work.

Now, I'm certainly not the only one to say this. In fact, if you browse the business section at your local book store you'll see a new trend in management-related books: an over-abundance of them speak to the importance of rest.

They suggest things like-

- Napping during the work day

- Getting 8 hours of sleep every night

- Optimal work weeks of no more than 36 hours

You read that last one right. *36 hours.* No typo there. In fact, multiple sources confirmed that after 36 hours of work you actually STOP producing and you simply begin coasting. There's no net gain.

Here's what got my attention: at 50-plus hours your work becomes a *negative.* That is, you actually begin undoing what you've done, thereby jeopardizing your progress from the week. Extra work doesn't get you ahead, it puts you in the hole. It "undoes" some of the great things you've achieved that week.

Think of it like this…

Athletes avoid over-training. They understand that there's an optimal amount of time and energy to expend on their physical progress. If they exert themselves too hard or train too long they don't provide enough time and space for their bodies to recover. They increase the likelihood of injury. In this case, more work isn't always better.

Another example…

Almost every morning I boil water to make instant coffee. I generally turn the knob on the stove and walk into the other room, collecting a few items and reviewing my schedule for the day. About twice a week I find myself so absorbed in my daily preview, though, that I *forget* about my water until I hear that slight singe that lets me know the last of my water is boiling off. When that happens, I'm forced to start the entire process over. More boiling isn't better; more boiling just does what's already been done.

A final example, the one from the cover of this book.

Look at those drums. In my opinion, no musician hustles on stage more than the drummer. Drummers keep the rhythm, they physically push their bodies, and they create a platform on which the rest of the band can play their music.

But (and this is important) music only happens *because of the moments of rest.* Watch the drummer next time. They're "not" playing more than they "are" playing. The rests are as important as the hits.

In fact, without the proper pauses, they just create noise. Rhythm is an acquired skill of maintaining the beat of times ON with a definite cadence of times OFF. The rests matter.

In the same way that good music depends on the times when the instruments are NOT being played, so also does life depend on the times when we're off. When we're still. When we're silent. And, this isn't just a new craze in business books or management fads. This is a principle that goes all the way back to Creation.

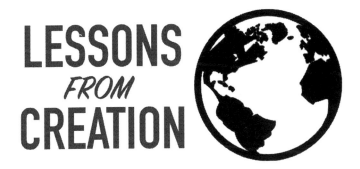

If you're like me, you consider your day to begin when you wake up in the morning. Right before you- if you're like me- prep that coffee. Or, if you stayed up to midnight, you may look at your watch and think, "Oh, gee… it's already tomorrow… a new day. I've got to get in bed."

We've programmed ourselves to think of our days as daylight first and then nighttime second. We get up and start the day; we go to bed and end it.

Turns out, *that's backwards*. We don't start each day's clock with the sun; we begin with the moon.

If you go all the way back to the beginning of the Bible, back to the very first page, you find the creation story. There, we read a refrain over and over and over again. It's so common that you may have never noticed it before. I guarantee you, though, once you see it, you'll never forget it.

Here it is: "There was evening and then morning, the _____ day."

We find it six times (Genesis 1:5,8,13,19,23,31). In God's rhythm of creation, days began with dark, not light. They began with the moon in the sky, not the sun. They began with sleep, not work. They began with rest, not activity.

SO THERE WAS EVENING AND THERE WAS MORNING- THE _____ DAY.

– Genesis 1:5,8,13,19,23,31

That's the rhythm of creation.

There's another example of this in the New Testament. Fast forward a few thousand years to the Cross. They removed Jesus from the Cross before sundown on Friday, the day He was executed, because Saturday was the Sabbath. Yet the Sabbath didn't begin on Saturday morning- or even at midnight. The Sabbath began at sundown, around 6pm (John 19:31). So, Friday at sundown they took Jesus from the Cross and placed Him in the tomb.

From the beginning, the new day began when the sun dropped, at sundown. That was the sign of a new day... *the rest.* The *rest* was first.

Let me show you something else that I hadn't noticed before I began diving into this "rest" thing: *when people were created.*

The Genesis story shows us that God created Adam at the *end* of Day 6. By the time the first man is scooped and formed from the dirt, God has been busy making all the animals that fill the earth (see Genesis 1:24). They were made on the same day, much earlier. Adam was created last, at the *end* of the 6th day.

Then came the seventh day.

Which began with evening (rest).

Which was followed by seventh morning (a complete 12 hours of daylight in which something new happened, something that had never been done before). God ordained that the entire day- every waking hour- would be one long *pause.*

This seventh day of rest was followed by the beginning of the eighth day which, of course, began with evening- more rest.

In other words, the first approximately 36-plus hours that Adam was alive were *full* of rest.

Let's add another layer to this. Read this verse.

THE LORD CAUSED A DEEP SLEEP TO FALL ON THE MAN, AND HE TOOK ONE OF HIS RIBS...

– Genesis 2:21

The story of Eve's creation is equally interesting. We learn that God creates her from the side of Adam. She's the crown of Creation (the final jewel that's displayed on the world), and she comes from the man.

The Bible uses a different word to describe how she was created than how Adam was made. Adam was "formed" from the dirt, a word in Hebrew used to describe what a common laborer might do when working with wood or clay. Eve, though, was "fashioned" from the man's rib, something more akin to creating a masterpiece or fine china (Genesis 2:22).

Paul tells us that "woman is the glory of man" (1 Corinthians 11:7). That is, when we see her glow, we can presume that the man has lived his calling- that he has promoted her, elevated her, and loved her well. He shines by causing her to radiate.

That said, take a look back at the story. *Where was Adam as this entire thing occurred?*

Yes, Adam slept- a deep sleep- through the entire process. That is, the greatest thing in which he ever participated happened while he rested.

Surely, there's a lesson in there for us, right? Multiple lessons, probably.

ON THE SEVENTH DAY HE RESTED FROM ALL THE WORK HE HAD MADE.

– Genesis 2:2

That said, we see a few rhythms present in creation:

First, each day starts with rest. This includes a cadence of rest and then work, rest and then work, rest and then work, rest and then work. But it *begins* with rest.

Second, each day of rest and work doesn't continue indefinitely. There's a 6 and 1, 6 and 1, 6 and 1, 6 and 1 beat in which the sixth day is always followed by a rest (night of day 7), rest (light of day 7), rest (night of day 1 of a new week).

We're made for this rhythm. And, when we step away from it...

We over-train and injure ourselves.

We boil the water off, undoing what's been done.

We beat, beat, beat, beat with no cadence and just create lives of noise.

Ready for some practical things you can do to step into this rhythm?

Here are three steps you take *NOW* to move away from the noise into this musical rhythm of creation.

First, sleep. You probably need *more* sleep than you're getting. A *lot more* of it.

Sleep is when your body rebuilds AND when your mind goes to rest and begins processing and mending and "figuring out" the stuff from your day. It's when you reset- completely.

Turns out, a lot of people AREN'T doing a daily- or even weekly reset.

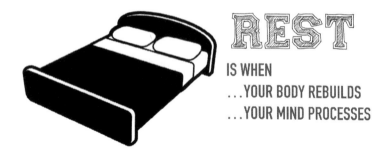

REST IS WHEN
...YOUR BODY REBUILDS
...YOUR MIND PROCESSES

This one is huge. Again business books are being written- not about mission or vision or the other things we typically attribute to biz- about getting more sleep. And about naps.

Why? Because in the same way your computer has to restart and recalibrate, so also do you.

There are 5 stages of sleep. Most people NEVER get out of that first bit where you're halfway asleep, halfway awake- that place where dreams and real life blur, the place where you keep waking up.

5 STAGES OF SLEEP

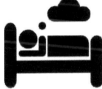

STAGE 1 BARELY ASLEEP (2-5%)
BLUR BETWEEN AWAKE & ASLEEP
ANXIETY KEEPS YOU HERE LONGER
NEVER GET TO DEEP SLEEP
GETS YOUR RHYTHM BACKWARDS

When you don't get enough rest, it flips things backwards. You start running on adrenalin at night (and can't sleep) and you begin crashing during the day.

Your body doesn't just need sleep when it's time to go to bed, though. Your body also needs rest when it's awake, too- space when you're not looking at your phone, occupying every minute.

When's the last time you day-dreamed? When's the last time your mind was free to wander... or wonder?

Same thing. When your mind is "free" it naturally makes the connections you need. (This explains why so many people receive their "best ideas" when they're exercising.)

DAY-DREAMING

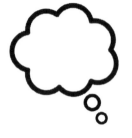

AT MENTAL REST
INNER BRAIN = 20X MORE ACTIVE!
INNER HEALING TAKES PLACE
WE- ODDLY ENOUGH- AVOID THIS
WE PREFER TO STAY "BUSY"

Here's the kicker.

Sleep experts studied people deprived of sleep and discovered that if you get less than 8 hours for 2 weeks in a row, you're operating at the same diminished capacity you would if you had too much to drink.

Except you haven't. And it's going on all day, every day.

Think about it.

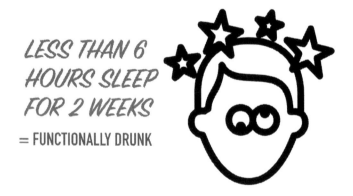

LESS THAN 6 HOURS SLEEP FOR 2 WEEKS
= FUNCTIONALLY DRUNK

Second, take a sabbath. Pick one day when you intentionally decide to just be present.

Adam and Eve weren't created to perform. They were made for *presence*.

The first thing that happens to them after they're made- in God's image- is that He speaks to them and blesses them (1:28). And then they go into their "day off."

The day was known as the Sabbath, and was a gift from God. It was, according to Jesus, made for us, so that we could reset (see Mark 2:27).

And so we can gain perspective.

And see that the important things in this life aren't things at all.

And experience the same gift that Adam & Eve received in Eden, the beauty of being present without performing.

Moses reminds us that God Himself rested and was refreshed from His work on the first Sabbath (Exodus 31:17). If He needed it- or, at least, embraced it- how much more should we?

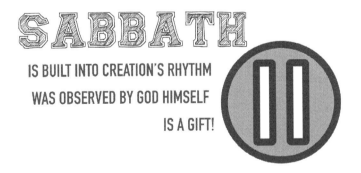

SABBATH

IS BUILT INTO CREATION'S RHYTHM

WAS OBSERVED BY GOD HIMSELF

IS A GIFT!

Third, seek the right things in the right way. Now, this one's important- so important that we're going to tackle it in the next chapter. My guess is that the reasons we often don't do #1 and #2 above are because we seek things- often the right things- in the wrong way.

Turn the page and I'll tell you more.

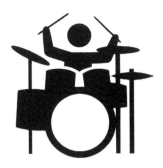

2. WHAT DOES IT MEAN TO SEEK THE RIGHT THINGS?

MAIN IDEA= IT'S NOT JUST THE THINGS WE SEEK- OR HUSTLE FOR- THAT MATTERS. RATHER, THE WAY IN WHICH WE HUSTLE IS IMPORTANT, TOO.

At the end of the previous chapter, I offered you three things you can do now to empower you to step into creation's rhythm and stop living with noise.

1. Sleep

2. Sabbath

3. Seek the right things in the right way

I hope you committed to scheduling the first two- that you....

First, actually wrote a bed time down- and committed to turning Netflix, your tablet, your smartphone, or any other thing off in order to get the rest your body needs.

(Remember, you should probably find a moment of pause during your day, as well- be it when you go for a run, a walk, a time of meditation, or some other moment when you embrace *presence* over *performance*.)

Second, you found a Sabbath. That is, you highlighted a full day during the week- one full 24-hour period- to unplug and just be present without performing.

In this chapter we'll talk about what it means to seek the right things. I promise, it's not what you think.

MY DESTINY DEPENDS ON MY HEALTH- NOT JUST MY HUSTLE

Here's where this chapter is headed:

Our ability to live our calling and reach our ultimate destiny (that dream for which we often strive) is dependent upon our health- not just our hustle. And health includes emotional wholeness, relational connectedness, spiritual well-being, and physical vitality. We must be healthy in order to maximize our effectiveness in all areas! We cannot reach our destiny if we're unhealthy or sick- *in any area of life.* This includes, particularly, the work of the soul.

(In the previous book in this series, *Emotional Wholeness Checklist*, we discussed the reality that many people overlook emotional health.)

I've learned that one of the biggest hindrances to walking with a healthy soul is striving, straining, and seeking to achieve things in my own strength. That is, it's not just "doing bad" things that knock us off course. Many times, we can do "good," but do it from a sense of obligation instead of overflow.

There's a great line in the Sermon on the Mount that speaks to this. I've placed it in the graphic below, emphasizing an important word.

(This chapter will be just like the last one. Even if you don't normally look to the Bible for guidance, stay with me for a few more pages. I guarantee you this will be super-insightful, too.)

> # "BUT SEEK FIRST THE KINGDOM OF GOD AND HIS RIGHTEOUSNESS, AND ALL THESE THINGS SHALL BE ADDED TO YOU."
>
> – Matthew 6:33

Matthew records Jesus' admonition: "*Seek* first His kingdom and His righteousness" (Matthew 6:33). Notice that word *seek*. It's important.

Jesus tells us that if we do this- if we seek His Kingdom first AND seek His righteousness- that "*all* these things will be added to you…"

What are the "these things" that Jesus is talking about?

Well, in this part of His teaching, He points to the grind of life. Everyone seeks food, clothing… the basics. He tells us not to worry about what we'll eat or what we'll wear.

"For after all these things the Gentiles *seek*," He says (Matthew 6:32).

Now, I used to think Jesus was just telling us, "Yeah. People in the world are anxious about the stuff of this world… they worry about things like…"

- The things they'll wear. Whether they'll look GQ or not. Whether it was made in a sweat shop, or whether a fair wage was paid to the workers.

- And the things they'll eat. Will there be enough to go around? Will it be gluten free? Is it organic or grass fed or does it have carcinogens or other random things that might hurt you in it?

- And everything else in life. Jobs. The kids' soccer practice. Dance recital. Traffic. The car. My goodness- the oil needs to be changed again. And we should really stop tossing money into repairs on the old one- it would be just as much to simply buy a new one with what we keep throwing down the drain at the auto shop?

In other words, I thought Jesus was just comparing what He's telling us to seek, as opposed to what most people seek.

Remarkably, though, it's not just the "object" of that search which He suggests should be different; it's also the manner of "seeking." You see, the word *seek* in this passage is two different words (in the Greek language) which we've translated as the same word in English.

- Jesus says *seek* "as a hunger, without labor or toil."

- The Gentiles *seek* "with much sweat, toil, stress, anxiety."

We could rephrase what Jesus tells us to do like this: "Hunger / desire (without labor or toil) for His kingdom and His righteousness… and everything else comes your way, too."

SEEKING MY DREAMS

"Gentiles" seek		Jesus says you seek
WITH MUCH SWEAT, TOIL, STRESS, ANXIETY	*VS.*	AS A HUNGER- WITHOUT LABOR OR TOIL

Do you see the difference?

- The seeking Jesus tells us to do is simply to desire… to trust… and to be prepared to receive.

- The seeking the world tells us to do is to, well… *toil*. We'll talk more about toil in chapter 5. Often, we confuse toil and hustle. They're *not* the same.

Jesus says, in effect, "My grace out-performs your default way of hustling. Rest in it. Stop *toiling*."

I thought about this the other day as I reflected on my kids. They wake up every morning and don't worry about a thing. Well, other than, "Hey, can we go do something fun…?" Or, "Can I have ANOTHER snack?!"

They don't wonder if there will be food in the pantry when they make their way from their bedrooms to the kitchen pantry.

I doubt they even know that there's such a thing as a power bill. Or a water bill. Or any kind of utilities.

In our house, the cars always run, the television always works, and the wifi- though it can drag a bit late in the evening when everyone in the neighborhood jumps on and starts binge-watching Netflix- seems to *always* work.

Notice-

- They don't "seek" these things. They just *desire* them.

- They don't *toil* for these. My grace to them delivers the goods.

In other words, they do the "first kind" of seek- not the second kind.

It's amazing that Jesus routinely calls us back to look at parent-child relationships in order to understand our Heavenly Father (i.e., Matthew 7:11). He says things like, "You know how this works… you do this… and IF YOU do this for your kids… HOW MUCH MORE will your Heavenly Father do this for you?"

Right?

- My resources are limited, His aren't.

- My love- let's be honest- has bounds. His doesn't.

- My patience… well… I'm still working on it. He, on other hand, is extremely patient and kind.

- And, whereas I'm subject to change moods with the emotional wave of the day, He is constant.

And, in light of this, He invites us to seek in the first way- not seek in the second way.

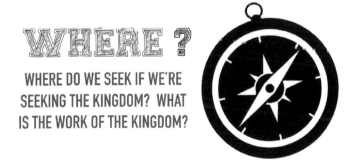

WHERE ?

WHERE DO WE SEEK IF WE'RE SEEKING THE KINGDOM? WHAT IS THE WORK OF THE KINGDOM?

So, how do we seek the kingdom? And how do we define the kingdom in a way that we can understand it and then actually do what Jesus says?

Paul actually defines the kingdom in the book of Romans: "The Kingdom of God is not a matter of eating and drinking, but righteousness and peace and joy in the Holy Spirit" (Romans 14:17).

If we join the two verses- Jesus' from the Sermon on the Mount (Matthew 6:33) and Paul's (Romans 14:17)- and exchange Paul's definitions for *kingdom* where Jesus mentioned "the kingdom," we get this:

- Seek first ~~the kingdom~~ *righteousness*… everything else comes.

- Seek first ~~the kingdom~~ *joy*… and everything else comes.

- Seek first ~~the kingdom~~ *peace*… and everything else comes.

That is…

- Desire righteousness… right relational connection with others.

- Desire joy… bliss, happiness, contentedness.

- Desire peace… harmony… honor.

When we do that, yes, everything else comes, too.

And, remember, the power to do this is always available, because Jesus said "the kingdom is among you" (Luke 7:28).

> **"THE KINGDOM OF GOD DOES NOT COME WITH OBSERVATION; NOR WILL THEY SAY, 'SEE HERE!' OR 'SEE THERE!' FOR INDEED, THE KINGDOM OF GOD IS WITHIN YOU."**
>
> – Luke 17:20-21

When you are spiritually vibrant, your entire outlook changes... you begin operating from the deepest part of you... everything is transformed. In other words, the starting point for seeking- for healthy hustling- isn't dreams or goals or vision boards. The starting line of healthy hustle is deep inside you.

And that leads us to chapter 3. We've got to know who we are or else we'll chase lesser things.

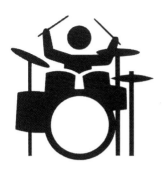

3. INTRINSIC IDENTITY

MAIN IDEA= A LOT OF HUSTLE IS A DESPERATE CHASE FOR SELF-WORTH. IF I DON'T RESOLVE WHO I AM- AND THAT I'M WORTHY. I'LL CHASE THAT VALUE IN EXTERNAL THINGS.

For many of us there always seems to be a gap between where we are now and where we want to be. And I'm not just talking about life "in general," *I'm talking about every specific area of life.*

No doubt, you've heard- *or even said-* things like this:

- I don't have enough money
- I don't have enough experience
- I don't have enough education

- I don't have enough sales

- I don't have enough time off from work

- I don't have enough time- *period*

All of these examples have one thing in common: *not enough.* That gap between where we are and where we want to be, between what we have and what we desire, is the "not enough" dilemma.

Why isn't there enough? Or, to be more "real" about it… why does there- from our perspective- always seem to be an *abundance* for everyone *except* for us?

The answer depends on the soundtrack you play in the background of your mind, doesn't it?

Well, we create the most clever reasons of all. We say things like:

- "I'm held back by my genetics."

- "I don't have enough education..."

- "I grew up in the wrong neighborhood."

- "My parents didn't give me the opportunities that..."

- "We don't have enough money..."

- "I'm the wrong race / gender / sexual orientation… people like me don't get the opportunities others get..."

Do you see what happens here?

First, we decide there's a lack of something. Since we're being honest, let's agree that there's usually a lack of several things- from our perspective, anyway.

(Whether or not something is lacking is another point entirely- something that we may also be able to resolve in this chapter.)

Second, we create a list of reasons *why* that lack exists. And it generally has to do with how *invaluable* we perceive ourselves to be, because of something we don't have.

Here's what I've learned from my own story. The soundtrack we tell ourselves is the reality we sell ourselves. And that reality becomes the one we live.

THE STORY WE TELL OURSELVES IS THE REALITY WE SELL OURSELVES

Humans are persistent, aren't we?

I mean, give us a problem (like a "not enough" issue) and we'll try to solve it. There wasn't enough land in Europe, so we entered the age of exploration and sent people all over the world on boats. There wasn't enough time to get from Point A to Point B, so we invented planes, trains, and automobiles. There's wasn't enough drama, so we concocted social media.

OK. I made up the last one.

Social media can be a great tool, right? But it can also lead to what we're talking about in this chapter... it can highlight that gap between where you are and where you want to be.

Besides, everyone displays the "greatest hits" version of their day online...

No one says, "Man, it's the end of the year. I missed my sales goals by 20%! #FailingForward #LearnByExperience #StillGrateful."

Nobody posts, "Our marriage is in the *for worst* part of our vows. Hoping to get to the *for better* part soon. #LoveIsForever #MarriageIsHard #PrayersPlease."

I've yet to see just one person confess, "Seeing all your great posts online makes me a bit jealous. Half of me is excited for you and half of me wonders when things will work out for me, too. #MixedEmotions #JustBeingHonest #TheStruggleIsReal."

See what I'm saying?

Anyway, after deciding that we lack something and after deciding that we'd be more valuable without that gap , here's what we do: *we most often insert someone or something into that gap to bridge the difference.* In other words, we do what humans have always done- we try to overcome the shortfall.

- We get married, thinking it will heal our hurts by making us feel loved.

- We seek to make more money, to acquire more stuff, or accumulate experiences everyone else wants. We often do this to show our value and worth, all by raising our socioeconomic status or changing our "status quo."

- We go to school, change careers, or seek new hobbies.

- We lose weight, gain weight, get new haircuts, go shopping, try new relationships, and (sometimes) even go under the knife.

Look back at the list. I want you to notice something. Two somethings, actually. Two somethings which are important.

First, none of these things are issues of right and wrong. To use Biblical language, none of them are sin. Sure, you can attempt to bridge your gap with sins- with drugs, rampant sex, or even gluttony (yeah, that one's in the Bible, too). However, although the things I listed above aren't "bad" in and of themselves, none of them can bring freedom. Though they may facilitate a temporary sense of relief, by themselves they're the equivalent of emotional band-aids. You can acquire any combination of these things- even all of them- and still lose your soul (see Luke 9:25).

Second, the items CAN WRONGLY BE rooted in identity- in who we are. It's easy to chase them because of some perceived need to supply something in the soul.

WHERE YOU ARE ISN'T WHO YOU ARE

About that second one…

Your Heavenly Father has already decided who you are, His beloved, the one in whom He's well pleased. No matter how great things are going or how bad they are, you're more than the sum of all your highest highs and certainly more valuable than the sum of all the deepest lows.

I'm an Alabama Fan. Roll Tide to the core.

Twenty five years ago the Tide won the National Championship under the leadership of Quarterback Jay Barker. (I know, that was *so many championships ago*, LOL!) That year, Barker led his team to demolish a much higher ranked, more favored Miami Hurricane squad. It so happened that the Hurricanes were also the defending champions.

Favored to win by *double digits*, the Hurricanes blew through the media circus like a storm. Players flaunted rings from their recent years of success. Others compared their speed to Alabama's. They openly trashed-talked on a level never seen on television before.

The sports commentators didn't help the situation much. They actually nagged it on.

And, one of their primary targets was the Alabama QB. They talked about how Barker could be in trouble. Did he measure up? Could his offensive line hold against the Hurricane defense? Would his team *even make it* the full 60 minutes of the game?

It sounds bizarre looking back, now that we know the end of the story. At the time, though, it's the soundtrack that was playing. Furthermore, almost everyone was listening. *Almost.*

One day on the radio, Barker revealed how he pushed through the media blitz.

"I never read the paper or watch you guys on TV," he told an announcer. This was before the day of the Internet and social media, by the way. He continued, "My Dad told me not to pay attention to you."

"Oh? Well, why not?" The interviewer was genuinely interested in what *that* might have to do with anything related to his success on the field.

"If I have a good game," Barker replied, "you guys overdue the praise. You give me credit for things that weren't even related to my performance- praise that should have gone to the offensive line, or to someone on defense who made a game-saving interception. When your words are kind, it's easy to think I'm better than I am…"

He continued, "When I have a bad game, you guys really pour it on. Even though I'm one of only a *few* starting quarterbacks in the *entire* nation, you can say things cruel enough to make me wonder how I ever got through Little League. It can be debilitating…"

He concluded, "I just don't listen to you guys, either way. I have a few people I trust- particularly my Coach and my Dad- and I let them keep me focused."

Boom.

That's kinda how *we* should be. We must know the source of our validation. Our darkest moments often deflate us- pushing us lower than we should ever be. And, on the other hand, our greatest hits moments can artificially inflate our identity to something we're not, to some false wonderland that's- get this- also less than who we really are.

A lot of us hustle in order to earn something that we already have. And that's why we become desperate- or feel inferior- when we don't achieve it. We're often chasing something that *hustle* can't supply. And why it often feels like toil.

A LOT OF HUSTLE IS A DESPERATE CHASE FOR SELF-WORTH

There's a story in the Bible that speaks to this.

One day the Pharisees and scribes found themselves frustrated with Jesus. Again. "This man receives sinners *and eats with them*," they said (see Luke 15:2).

They were infuriated. Disgusted. Appalled.

Eating was important. Anytime you ate with anyone you were pledging yourself to them in some significant way. It was an act of covenant loyalty.

That's why the Pharisees *often* asked, "Why does your teacher eat with tax collectors and sinners?"

In response, Jesus told them the story we've come to know as the "Prodigal Son." You may remember it. It's the parable about a father and his two grown sons. The youngest decides he wants his inheritance early, so he asks his father for it in full (this was an insult, by the way, the equivalent of wishing the father dead).

Over the next season of life, he squanders his money, losing *everything*. Penniless, he decides to return home, rationalizing that he can serve as a "hired hand" in the fields of his father. At least then he'll have somewhere to go, something to do with his life. He's content to *toil* for his room and board.

You know the end of *his* part of the tale. The father sees him returning from afar (because he's been watching and waiting, hoping for him to come back!). He breaks social custom and runs to his son (gentlemen didn't run in public).

He gives his son a robe, a signet ring, and sandals- demonstrating that the younger boy remains a son (robe), he retains his authority (ring), and he's trusted to come and go from the estate as he pleases (shoes).

According to Old Testament law, the son should have been stoned for his rebellion (Deuteronomy 21:18-21). The father is actually the one who should have brought the charge. Rather than doing this, though, the father does something extraordinary. He throws a party. He kills the fatted calf, because his son- who was "dead"- has come home.

Now for the rest of the story, the part related to toil…

The older brother hears the dancing and singing from this celebration as he labors in the fields. As he approaches the estate, he asks the servants about the commotion.

"Your brother has returned," they tell him. "Your father killed the prize calf and is throwing a big party!"

When Jesus communicates the story, He says the older brother gets *angry* about this. He *refuses* to attend the party (15:28).

Now, let's step back and pause. *Let's remember why Jesus launched into this tale in the first place.* Remember, He has a cadre of religious elitists who've been following all of the rules, watching others squander the estate (by tax collecting and sinning), and wondering why Jesus dared cozy up to them.

They've been toiling- in the religious sense. Life has been one unhealthy hustle- all in the name of maintaining the status quo and shoring up their identity.

This stance was compounded by the fact that centuries earlier Moses taught the people that if they followed God's rules they would be able to live in the Promised Land forever. If they didn't, they'd be exported from the land and/or enslaved by others who would rule over them (see Deuteronomy 28).

Most of the Pharisees knew enough of their nation's history to realize that this seemed to be how things worked. Their ancestors experienced the period of the Judges in which they were beaten ruthlessly, their great-great-great-great grandparents had been sacked by the Assyrians and Babylonians, and they had seen the Temple destroyed and rebuilt....

Even now, these Pharisees (and Jesus) lived under Roman occupation, enduring heavy taxation and over-bearing oppression. They *knew* what it was like to *not* be free. Moreover, many of them believed that strict obedience to the Old Testament law would create an environment where God could move and thrust off their oppressors, thereby bringing an age of the Kingdom of God.

The more Jesus embraced "sinners," the more He seemed to thwart this! He was encouraging the very people who were keeping God's blessings *away* from the nation, they reasoned! This was a point of high contention between them and

Jesus. And, remember, Jesus is telling them *this story* to answer why He "entertains" the very ones whose disobedience seems to be the cause of their ongoing calamity.

Notice the parallels: in the same way the Pharisees refuse to come near to God (Jesus is God in the flesh)- because of the "rift-raft" people hanging close to God, the older brother refuses to go near his father because of the squanderer that's near him. *This stance effectively keeps the older brother- and the Pharisees- at a distance from the One who's inviting them to stop toiling, to cease finding their identity in the externals, and come in close...*

What happens next in the story is amazing. The father breaks *another* social norm- he leaves the banqueting table at his own party.

I imagine he offered the same grace as he sought this older son, too.

"Come inside," the father says, as he finds his son amidst his toil.

However, the older brother puts distance between him and his father because he can't reconcile the grace that's been offered to the younger son.

He says, "This son *of yours* has returned... and you've killed the calf."

He doesn't say, "This brother *of mine* is back" (15:29).

He can't stand the fact that they're related to one another, right?

He even points out issues in his father's behavior- much like the Pharisees tried to poke holes in Jesus' choice of relationships.

"You never gave me a party?!" The older son says. "All the years that I never disobeyed and you never offered me a young goat so I could celebrate with my friends!"

The father, in love, looks at his oldest son. He tells him plainly: "Everything I have is yours" (Luke 15:31).

And- "It always has been."

In other words, the older son has been toiling for something he already possessed!

Remember what the younger brother planned to do? Yes, go work in the field, as a servant, earning his keep.

And where do we find the older brother while the party happens? Yes, in the field... which, *in his mind,* earns his keep.

"EVERYTHING I HAVE IS ALREADY YOURS."

– Luke 15:31

You can imagine the scribes saying something like this to Jesus. "Why do You dine with tax collectors and sinners?" Then- "Why don't You commune with us? After all, we've earned it. We're doing everything right."

That's the follow-up question, isn't it? And it's why they think they're worthy... they've been toiling.

It's also why Jesus repeatedly tells them, "Those who are well have no need of a physician" (see Luke 5:31).

Or, to say it another way- "You're well. You don't need the doctor."

And- "I've not come to call the righteous, but sinners" (Mark 2:17).

You can almost see Jesus *commending* them when you read things from this perspective. I mean, in other verses He actually boasts about their righteousness (see Matthew 5:20, 23:23)?

Furthermore, I imagine Jesus would say to those same Pharisees, "Hey, I'd love for you to come into this party, too- the one with the tax collectors and sinners and harlots and others… You don't have to change who you are to come inside… You just need to accept them for who they are… And you've got to stop toiling. You can't attend the party and work in the field at the same time, because it's impossible to be in two places at once."

Perhaps this is why He looked at a group of religious zealots one day and said, "Harlots and tax collectors enter the Kingdom ahead of you" (Matthew 21:31).

It's not that the Pharisees weren't welcome, it's just that they were "older-brothering" it. They wouldn't "go in" if "less desirable" people were already at the party. So, like the older brother, they kept working in the field. They continued serving God with the tiniest minutia of the Law, even toiling the smallest things like tithing the spices in their kitchen cabinet (Matthew 23:23).

Again, the father in Jesus' story reminds the older brother that he has *always* had access to the entire estate (15:31). As such, he could have taken a goat and celebrated anytime he wanted to. He can't see that, though, because in the end he really believes some of the things that we wrongly believe:

- Following all of the rules is what gives us favor with the Father (and not following them should exclude others from that favor), *and*

- We often (wrongly) believe that we enter the Father's estate by grace- through no effort of our own. But then we have to work and "prove" that we deserve to be there, effectively putting ourselves back in the position of toiling servants instead of sons and daughters.

The truth is that both boys were focused on themselves and their part of the estate. They just expressed it in different ways. One squandered; the other toiled. Both found their identity in their "stuff" instead of the relationship .

This means that, for the older brother, the moment of repentance would have been *to do the exact same thing as the younger brother-* stop seeing himself as a servant and embrace the fact that he is- and always has been- a son. In other words, put on the robe, the ring, and the shoes… *and to stop fighting to earn what's been freely offered.*

Does this mean we don't work? Does it mean we don't venture into the fields?

Quite the opposite. We do. But, when we work, we hustle in healthy ways instead of unhealthy ways. Turn the page and I'll explain.

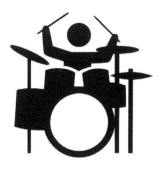

4. HOLY HUSTLE

MAIN IDEA= ANY WORK CAN BE SACRED; ANY HUSTLE CAN BE HOLY. WHAT'S THAT MEAN? QUITE SIMPLY, IT'S RESERVED FOR SOMETHING SPECIAL.

After reviewing the previous chapter you might be thinking, "Oh, wow. It seems like he's arguing against work."

Ummm... no.

Just the opposite. In fact, let me show you how the Bible presents "work."

Quite simply this: work isn't a result of the Fall. God gave Adam and Eve stewardship of the entire planet before sin and chaos ever entered the equation. Check it for yourself. They were given stewardship of the planet in Genesis 1:28. Toil doesn't enter until Genesis 3:17- two full chapters later.

In the beginning, they didn't work to bolster their identity or self-worth, like we discussed in the previous chapter, they knew who they were…

And they didn't work in the sense of toiling. Work was a gift, a means they used to add value to the world around them. Through their work, they co-created with God, making things better for everything in the created order.

WORK ISN'T A RESULT OF THE FALL- TOIL IS

And notice, none of their work was necessarily "spiritual" in the sense that we think of spiritual work. They weren't preaching or leading Bible studies. They were overseeing the planet, exercising dominion over the animals, and building a family. Yet it was *all* sacred and valuable.

Think about that for a moment.

There's a tendency in the church to view "full time ministry" as *more spiritual* work and "full time something else" as *less spiritual.* We even suggest that those who work in the church full time are "called"- the obvious flip side being that those who don't simply aren't.

We've created a false dichotomy, a hierarchy the Bible doesn't create. Thankfully, the church is swinging the pendulum back to the middle, upholding the truth that people can be *called* to do all sorts of things. That is, a teacher can be just as called as a pastor who can be no more called than a fireman who can be just as called as an evangelist.

A true story from the trenches...

A few years ago I taught about healing at a church. I actually taught most of the content from one of the books in this series, *Health + Healing and Essential Oils*. I taught it on a Sunday morning, during the worship service. At the end of our time together, I invited people to come receive prayer if they had a physical issue they wanted to see remedied.

After praying for a few dozen people, I noticed a young woman wanting prayer. I invited her to come speak to me.

"I feel like God wants me to heal people, too," she offered.

She said it reluctantly, though, like she was holding back some of the info.

"Tell me about yourself," I replied. "What do you like to do...?"

"I'm about to finish school," she said. "I'm in college. I've got a family and I've been working on my degree for a few years... we've all made sacrifices so that I can finish, but I feel like I'm supposed to be healing people with God's power, with His touch... like you talked about."

She explained that she was ready to work, and that her family needed the income. They'd sacrificed for years in order for her to push through school. Now, she felt this tension between doing what God called her to do while having just taken a (costly) run at school for several years and now needing to help with the family finances.

"What's your degree?" I asked.

"Nursing."

"Nursing?" I replied. "Do you enjoy it?"

She told me she did. But, somehow she felt she was supposed to be healing people.

"Does it feel like *toil* when you do it?" I asked. "Or does it feel energizing and life-giving."

She smiled and told me- *shyly at first-* that she loved it. But, in her words, a church leader insinuated that if she was really following the call of God for her life she would pursue ministry full time. She'd get her degree and never show up for work as a nurse.

I explained to her that, in my opinion, she had chosen the *perfect* profession for a healer. "Where else are you going to have access to people at their most vulnerable moments? Where else do people need a touch? I mean… you're going to be with people and their families when they are sick and desperate… when things seem hopeless… and you're going to be able to carry your light there…"

I told her that she could pray for them. Even if sometimes it had to just be silent, it would still work…

"And the medicine and technology you'll have access to," I added, "It's all God's, anyway. And He has it there for you…"

After about 60 seconds of coaching her through this, she got it. She looked lighter. She began smiling again. She left feeling empowered… and called…

That's what *vocation* means, right? The root of the word, *vocal*, means to hear the voice… the calling… over what you do. And you can hear that voice telling you to do anything.

Think back to what we've learned over the past few pages:

- There's a rhythm to creation, and things work better when we live in it, savoring the moments of pause (chapter 1)

- We seek the best things not by striving for them but by hungering for them (chapter 2)

- Our identity is intrinsic to who we are- it's not external, so we'll never find it by hustling (chapter 3)

Once we understand those three ideas, we're free to work as on overflow of who we are. And, at this point, we see that *any* work can be sacred, and any hustle can be holy.

(By the way, *holy* is a great word. It means, "set apart for something special or sacred." And that's what our work becomes- something that doesn't give us value but something we use to impart value to the world around us, just like Adam and Eve were blessed to do in Genesis 1:28.)

ANY WORK CAN BE SACRED— ANY HUSTLE CAN BE HOLY

Dan Miller wrote a book, *48 Days to the Work You Love*, in which he pushes people to pursue that voice- that calling. He reminds us that in the Biblical mindset from which Jesus lived, there was no distinction as to who was called and who wasn't…

Anyone could hear the voice and follow…

He writes,

"THERE IS A HEBREW WORD, AVODAH, FROM WHICH COME BOTH THE WORDS "WORK" AND "WORSHIP." TO THE HEBREW MAN, HIS THURSDAY MORNING ACTIVITIES WERE JUST AS MUCH AN EXPRESSION OF WORSHIP AS BEING IN THE SYNAGOGUE ON THE SABBATH…"

– Dan Miller, 48 Days

"NOTHING IN SCRIPTURE DEPICTS THE CHRISTIAN LIFE AS DIVIDED INTO SACRED AND SECULAR PARTS. RATHER, IT SHOWS A UNIFIED LIFE, ONE OF WHOLENESS, IN WHICH EVERYTHING WE DO IS SERVICE TO GOD, INCLUDING OUR DAILY WORK, WHATEVER THAT MAY BE."

– Dan Miller, 48 Days

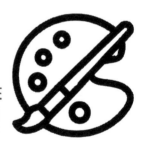

This isn't just a "spiritual concept," though- this idea about work being connected to a deeper purpose. Webster's dictionary (full disclosure: I looked this up online and not from an actual Webster's book!) defines work as "bodily or mental efforts exerted to do or make something; purposeful activity."

According to the dictionary, then, *work* is-

- Purposeful

- Meaningful

- Intentional

In fact, if it's not those adjectives, then it's not work at all, right? It's just… toil.

IF I FIND MY VALUE IN THE THINGS I DO, I'LL NEVER STOP HUSTLING

Once you're on the performance cycle, hustling to earn your value, you're stuck… doomed to continually run the treadmill (unless you jump off and stop playing the game).

The performance cycle is simply the religious version of the Eagles' *Hotel California*. "You can check in, but you can never leave." Unless you just quit playing and jump out the window, that is.

In the next chapter I'll tell you *why* you need to jump off. Whereas work is divine, toil is downright evil.

Sounds like an over-statement I know. Flip the page, and I'll explain.

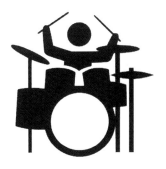

5. TOIL IS EVIL / WORK IS DIVINE

MAIN IDEA= HUSTLE CAN EASILY BECOME TOIL. THE OPPOSITE OF WORK ISN'T LAZINESS. THE OPPOSITE OF WORK IS TOIL. HUSTLE, BUT HUSTLE IN A HEALTHY WAY.

In chapter 4 we decided that all work can be holy, that any hustle can be sacred. We're created- and called- to add value to the world around us.

Now, let's add a final layer to this discussion.

The opposite of "work" isn't laziness, it's toil. And toil is that sense of striving and laboring that lacks purpose, lacks meaning, and lacks eternal intention.

Think back to what we learned in the previous chapter.

Work is not simply "punching in" and "punching out," passing through hours on a time clock, exchanging time spent doing something you don't want for the money that you need.

- If you hate your work, you're not really working. *You're toiling.* True work flows from something you love.

- If your work is disconnected from the life of the Spirit, you're not really working. *That's toil*, too. True work is totally connected to *worship*, however it is that you define that term.

- If your work lacks purpose, you're doing a "job," instead of living a calling. In other words, *more toil.*

Remember, true work is not a result of the Fall, but *toil* is. Work was given to Adam and Eve well before sin entered the equation- to serve as a process for them to steward creation and add value to the world around them- a world that was already very, very good.

THE OPPOSITE OF WORK ISN'T "LAZINESS."
THE OPPOSITE OF WORK IS UNBRIDLED HUSTLE, TOIL.

The Apostle John wrote the Gospel of John, the Book of Revelation, and 3 letters to his church (1 John, 2 John, 3 John). The verse in the graphic at the bottom of this page is the way he "signs off" his first letter, warning them- and us- to stay away from idols.

If you read the entire letter (it will take you less than 15 minutes), you'll notice that this seems like a super-strange ending to the entire message. You see, I always thought John was about the counterpoints of things like-

- Light vs. dark

- Love vs. not loving

- The works of Jesus vs. the works of the devil

However, after making these comparisons, John ends things- seemingly abruptly- with a conclusion that we should stay away from idols.

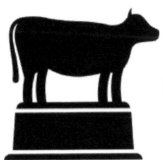

"LITTLE CHILDREN, GUARD YOURSELVES FROM IDOLS."
1 John 5:21

What gives?! Well, turns out, the verses just above this conclusion give us a clue as to what he might mean here.

In 1 John 5:19, just two sentences earlier than this warning about idols, John says, "We are of God, but the world lies under the power of the evil one."

On the surface, that sounds like a logical statement. And, we could even put these two verses together to make a statement like this: "There are evil influences in the world, so don't make any idols out of any of them."

Let's go deeper, though.

Strong's Concordance sheds some light on this passage. In this verse "evil one" is better translated as "the toil." That's right. Our Bible translators went to the obvious- "the world is evil."

But John offers us a more subtle message. He's telling us that the world is under the influence of- get this- *toil*. That's right, "The whole world lies under the power of [toil]" (1 John 5:19).

Or, to say it another way, "The world is under the power of unhealthy hustle, of striving, of the wrong kind of seeking."

John isn't just showing us a juxtaposition between us and "the world" (when did Christian become some anti-"the world," anyway?). He's highlighting something else we all know that we want to steer clear of... *toil*.

Who likes toil? None of us.

What exactly is toil? Well, to toil is...

- to work extremely hard, incessantly
- to drag, to struggle

- to strive, that is, to seek in the "first kind of seek" we discussed in chapter 2

In his book, *Money & the Prosperous Soul*, Steven DeSilva says that toil is "an oppressive force that separates work from its intended purpose."

He then does an interesting- and enlightening- exercise. He observes, "Notice what happens if we exchange the words *evil one* with *toil* in other common verses."

- "When anyone hears the word of the kingdom and does not understand it, ~~the evil one~~ *toil* comes and snatches away what was sown in his heart" (Matthew 13:19).

- "The field is the world, the good seeds are the sons of the kingdom, but the tares are the sons of ~~the evil one~~ *toil*" (Matthew 13:38).

- "I do not pray that you should take them out of the world, but that you should keep them from ~~the evil one~~ *toil*" (John 17:15).

- "Above all, take the shield of faith with which you will be able to quench all the fiery darts of ~~the evil one~~ *toil*" (Ephesians 6:16).

- "But the Lord is faithful, who will establish you and guard you from ~~the evil one~~ *toil*" (2 Thessalonians 3:3).

- "I have written to you, young men, because you are strong, and the word of God abides in you, and you have overcome ~~the evil one~~ *toil*" (1 John 2:13-14).

- "We know that whoever is born of God does not sin; but he who has been born of God keeps himself, and ~~the evil one~~ *toil* does not touch him" (1 John 5:18).

Here's the verse from John's letter again-

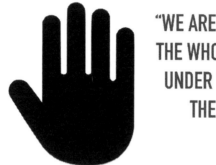

"WE ARE OF GOD, & THAT THE WHOLE WORLD LIES UNDER THE POWER OF THE ~~EVIL ONE.~~ *TOIL*

1 John 5:19

What are the most important takeaways?

Well, notice Ephesians 6:16 from DeSilva's list on the previous page: faith and trust actually shield us from toiling- from rushing to the tyranny of doing everything, and of being able to (instead) focus on the things that matter most.

When we trust our Father, and when we rest in the identify He gifts us… and step into the restful rhythm of His creation…

When we lean into the heart of our Heavenly Father we get a sense of, "He's got this… we don't have to strive for it… No more toiling…"

Or, "Hustle, but hustle in a healthy way…"

That is-

- Hustle with a definite rhythm of on and off- one that has more off than on (chapter 1)

- Hustle by hungering for Me and the things I want to shower upon you, not as a striving and chasing of the wind (chapter 2)

- Hustle as an overflow of the gifts and calling I've placed in you- not to earn something you already have (chapter 3)

- Hustle to bless others, to add value, to steward creation and make this place better for everyone (chapter 4)

Once we get that perspective, it's interesting that the final phrase of 1 John is "keep yourselves from idols…"

It's easy for us to fill our schedules- toiling, chasing things, seeking after stuff that was never part of God's design for us- things that were never part of our "how" to begin with.

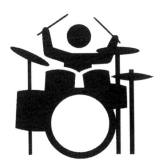

6. TEN MUST HAVE OILS FOR LIFE BALANCE

MAIN IDEA= TWO OILS FROM EACH TOPIC TO ENCOURAGE, EQUIP + EMPOWER YOU TO WALK IN YOUR TRUE IDENTITY AND TO STEP FROM TOIL INTO HEALTHY HUSTLE.

In the first five chapters of the book we explored several themes:

- Chapter 1 = Rest (the rhythm of creation), including sleep and pausing throughout the day

- Chapter 2 = Seeking (being present) vs. striving (performing)

- Chapter 3 = Identity, understanding your value is in who you are NOT in what you do or where you stand in relation to your goals

- Chapter 4 = Stewardship and healthy hustle, as we're all called to do something extraordinary- as an overflow of who we already are

- Chapter 5 = Embracing the future as a gift, not as something for which we toil

We've selected ten oils- 2 for each theme. The first two were chosen for chapter 1, the second two for chapter 2, etc.

Over the next few pages we'll describe each, why to use them, and how to apply. For more information on the science behind the oils, visit OilyApp.com and login to the March 2019 edition of OilyApp+, entitled *Healthy Hustle*.

TEN MUST HAVE OILS FOR LIFE BALANCE

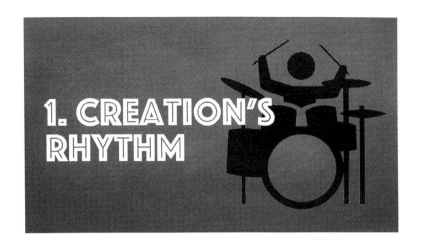

1. CREATION'S RHYTHM

MAIN IDEA= IN MUSIC, THE RESTS ARE AS IMPORTANT AS THE NOTES YOU PLAY. LIFE IS THE SAME WAY. THERE'S A DEFINITE BEAT TO CREATION THAT WORKS WELL FOR US WHEN WE EMBRACE IT.

GOALS=

- SLEEP 8 HOURS PER NIGHT. SCHEDULE IT NOW AS A "TEST RUN" FOR A SOLID WEEK. AT THE END OF THE 7 NIGHTS OF SLEEPING MORE, ASSESS HOW YOU FEEL. ADJUST UP OR DOWN AFTER THAT AS NEEDED.

- PAUSE DURING THE DAY. GIVE YOURSELF TIME TO REFLECT. BY MAKING SPACE FOR EXERCISE, FOR THINKING AND DREAMING, FOR MEDITATION AND/OR PRAYER.

- BE "ON" WHEN YOU'RE WORKING, AND COMPLETELY "OFF" WHEN YOU'RE OFF. NO SNEAK-PEAKS AT THE CELL PHONE, NO CHECKING EMAIL, ETC.

- "CHECK OUT" OF EVERYTHING- EXCEPT FOR OFF-LINE RELATIONSHIPS (PHONING YOUR FAMILY + FRIENDS TO ACTUALLY TALK ABOUT NON-WORK-RELATED ISSUES = OK) FOR ONE 24-HOUR PERIOD EACH WEEK.

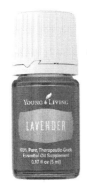

PAUSE

1
2-3 DROPS
OF EACH
YOUNG LIVING
ESSENTIAL OIL

2 APPLY TO TEMPLES,
WRISTS + HANDS + HEART

LAVENDER

Our natural tendency is to do things in our own strength, with our steam. We chug along with the best mental talk we can muster- "I think I can, I think I can, I think I can... I...."

Nothing against positivity. Let's be real. We need more of it.

The Bible even tells us, "As you think... so are you..." (Proverbs 23:7)

At the same time, get this: the same grace that saves you is the same grace that empowers you to fulfill your destiny (see Ephesians 2:8-10)

Can you achieve in the flesh the thing that God began in the Spirit (Galatians 3:3)? The answer is no...

Live in the rhythm of creation. Don't strive. Pause.

It's this grace that saves, mends, forgives, empowers, heals, imparts, encourages...

... and we need reminders of it throughout the day.

For the next 30 days, take a few breaks during your work week. Schedule them now- perhaps even by setting reminders in your calendar. Five or ten minutes.

Use Lavender to enhance relaxation and hit your personal pause button.

DEEP SLEEP

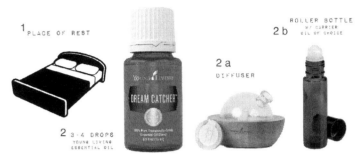

1 PLACE OF REST

2 3-4 DROPS
YOUNG LIVING
ESSENTIAL OIL

2 a
DIFFUSER

ROLLER BOTTLE
W/ CARRIER
OIL OF CHOICE
2 b

DREAM CATCHER

You need more sleep. A lot more of it.

Sleep is when your body rebuilds AND when your MIND goes to rest and begins processing and mending and "figuring out" the stuff from your day. It's when you reset- completely.

Turns out, a lot of people AREN'T doing a daily- or even weekly reset.

This one is huge. So big, in fact, that business books are being written- not about mission or vision or the other things we typically attribute to biz- about getting more sleep. And about naps.

Why? Because in the same way your computer has to restart and recalibrate, so also do you.

There are 5 stages of sleep. Most people NEVER get out of that first bit where you're halfway asleep, halfway awake. That place where dreams and real life blur. That place where you keep waking up.

When you don't get enough rest, it flips things backwards. You start running on adrenalin at night (can't sleep) and you begin crashing during the day.

Your body needs rest when it's awake, too- space when you're not looking at your phone, occupying every minute. When's the last time you day-dreamed? Same thing. It's a time when your mind wanders, makes the connections you need, and works forward.

Here's the kicker. They studied people who lacked sleep and discovered that if you get less than 8 hours for 2 weeks in a row, you're operating at the same diminished capacity you would if you had too much to drink. Except you haven't. And it's going on all day, every day.

Think about it.

And then diffuse your Dream Catcher, rub some on the bottom of your feet, lay back... and chill.

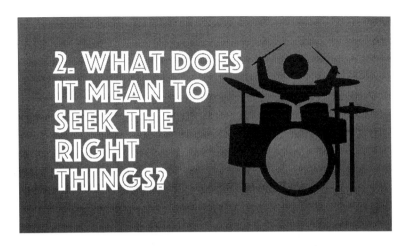

MAIN IDEA= IT'S NOT JUST THE THINGS WE SEEK- OR HUSTLE FOR- THAT MATTERS. RATHER, THE WAY IN WHICH WE HUSTLE IS IMPORTANT, TOO.

GOALS=

· EVALUATE WHETHER YOU SEEK (IN THE SENSE JESUS TALKED ABOUT) OR WHETHER YOU STRIVE. BE HONEST WITH YOURSELF.

· DOES STRESS, ANXIETY, OR WORRY CAUSE YOU TO LEAVE THE GRACE OF SEEKING... AND JUMP INTO STRIVING?

· HOW CAN YOU RECALIBRATE AND REFOCUS?

· HOW CAN YOU PLAN NOW TO HANDLE STORMS THAT WILL COME LATER?

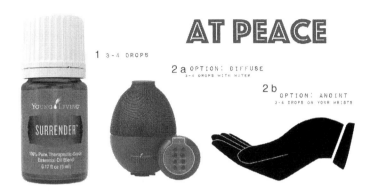

SURRENDER

Do the deeper work of the soul.

It's the only work that actually works. Everything else… is just a chasing after the wind, right?

The Scripture shows me that God can be found in our emotions. And that seeking the Kingdom often involves not simply doing things out in the world but also in doing the tough, deep work of the soul. That means exploring what's happening inside- and uncovering why.

Here's what I mean…

James says to "Count it all joy when you endure trials" (James 1:2). I historically assumed he referred only to the external pressure we face. Perhaps he does. But, the reality is that externals most often place weight on the soul.

I do know that James promises something to those who endure the dark night. In James 1:3-4, he says to consider it joy…

> *"because you know that the testing of your faith produces perseverance. Let perseverance finish its work so that you may be mature and complete, not lacking anything."*

Yes. In the end, we emerge complete. Whole. Better.

It sucks. But it fits with the promise that God uses all things for our good (Romans 8:28). NOT that all things ARE good. Some are horrible. Some aren't fair.

But… there's a tension here…

In the tension, God takes us to the "end" of ourselves, to a place where we can no longer rely on our personal resources. At that point, He takes us to a place where He produces something *new* and *substantial* inside us.

But, it only works if you do the deep work. If you don't band-aid it. Don't short-cut it…

If you dig…

SURRENDER

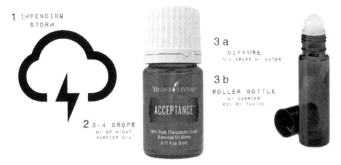

1 IMPENDING
STORM

3 a
DIFFUSE
3-4 DROPS W/ WATER

3 b
ROLLER BOTTLE
W/ CARRIER
OIL OF CHOICE

2 3-4 DROPS
W/ OR W/OUT
CARRIER OIL

ACCEPTANCE

Storms come. That's reality.

But, did you know…? YOU are in control of your emotions. And those emotions can serve you, OR not serve you. They can help you, OR they can hinder you.

The book Emotional Intelligence 2.0 reports that people with the highest IQs outperform people with lower IQs only 20% of the time- yet people with higher EQs (emotional quotients) out-perform higher IQs over 70% of the time.

EQ accounts for a pay increase of $28K per year- across all fields.

EQ can be learned. You can GROW in your emotional quotient.

How? By learning to recognize your emotions when they happen… then STOPPING to read what they're saying BEFORE you respond.

It's a mark of health, and it will serve you- and those around you- incredibly well.

Here's a go-to: Acceptance.

When you feel overloaded, step back, pause, and apply to your wrists and/or back of your neck. Or diffuse.

Breathe deep, and think about what's happening, what's going on inside of you.

Don't react. Give yourself 15 minutes before doing ANYTHING. Talk yourself down…

Then respond in a healthy way.

Repeat. Repeat. Repeat.

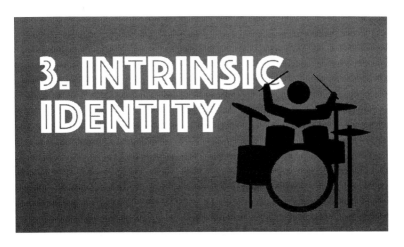

3. INTRINSIC IDENTITY

MAIN IDEA= A LOT OF HUSTLE IS A DESPERATE CHASE FOR SELF-WORTH. IF I DON'T RESOLVE WHO I AM- AND THAT I'M WORTHY, I'LL CHASE THAT VALUE IN EXTERNAL THINGS.

GOALS=

· TAKE AN HONEST LOOK AT WHY YOU WANT TO ACHIEVE THE GOALS YOU WANT TO ACHIEVE. ARE THEY BENCHMARKS? OR ARE THEY SOMETHING MORE? OR THEY TRULY AN OVERFLOW OF WHO YOU ARE- OR, ARE THEY SOMETHING TO SERVE AS AN INFLOW- TO PROVIDE VALUE TO YOU?

· ASK YOUR CLOSEST FRIENDS TO ASSESS THIS FOR YOU. MAKE SURE THEY HAVE THE FREEDOM TO BE HONEST WITHOUT FEAR OF REPERCUSSION OR RELATIONAL PUNISHMENT FROM YOU.

· NOTICE HOW MANY TIMES IN THE BIBLE JESUS SEEMS UN-HURRIED. HE LITERALLY HAS 3 YEARS TO SAVE THE ENTIRE WORLD, ALL HUMANITY FOR ALL TIME... AND HE NEVER RUSHES. AS A RESULT, MANY OF HIS MIRACLES ARE "INTERRUPTIONS" THAT HE CAN TAKE, BECAUSE HE HAS MARGIN. THE WOMAN WITH THE FLOW OF BLOOD, THE MAN WHO WAS LOWERED THROUGH THE ROOF BY HIS FRIENDS... THE FEEDING OF THE 5,000... AND

SO MANY MORE OF HIS MIRACLES WERE INSTANCES WE WOULD
INTERPRET- IN OUR WORLD- AS KINKS IN THE SCHEDULE. STEP BACK
AND RESOLVE HOW NOT CHASING FOR YOUR IDENTITY EMPOWERS YOU
TO SLOW DOWN AND STEP INTO A RHYTHM THAT ALLOWS YOU TO
SERVE OTHERS IN UNIQUE WAYS, USING YOUR OWN SKILLS + ABILITIES.

· WHAT AREAS OF YOUR LIFE NEED RESTORATION? ARE THESE AREAS IN
WHICH IT WOULD BE WORTH A BIT OF HUSTLE?

♕ KINGS & QUEENS

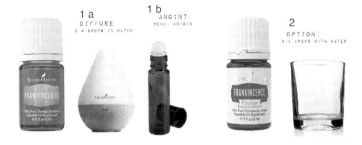

1 a
DIFFUSE
3-4 DROPS IN WATER

1 b
ANOINT
NECK, WRISTS

2
OPTION:
3-4 DROPS WITH WATER

FRANKINCENSE

One of the most popular oils throughout history. It was used to infuse the tabernacle AND the temple in the Old Testament... and is 1 of the 3 gifts the Magi delivered to Mary + Joseph + Jesus.

It was so widely known in those days that they commonly referred to it as "incense." Say the second part of the word and it was a GIVEN that you meant to add the first part. It was to essential oils what Coke is to soda... it was synonymous.

Yet this oil was super-special.

It was THE oil they used to anoint the newborn sons of Kings & Queens... meaning... people who would one day walk in their destiny as Kings & Queens themselves.

The great ones.

The ones like you.

Feeling blue? Then go with this red.

Transcend the emotional gap between what you *feel to be true and what you *know to be true. That there's more for you, that you're destined for more.

And get that revelation deep inside of you- into the deep, hidden parts of your brain (pic 2, 3), where revelation and sensory input come… where you connect with the greatness of the Kingdom.

Because you're a King. Or a Queen.

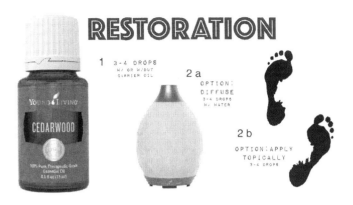

CEDARWOOD

Lepers were given Cedarwood, as they were healed and restored to the faith community.

Why? Because Cedarwood enhances mental sharpness. And, it helps them re-align with the truth of their identify: restored, whole, complete.

The beams in the temple were constructed of Cedarwood (1 Kings 4:33, Psalm 104:15), likely to assist people in learning AND in knowing how they are as they walked in to worship.

The oil also assists with emotional cleaning and release.

As you contemplate who you are- that you are enough (with or without your accomplishments, with or without any externals)- use Cedarwood. Diffuse it, place it on your feet (as the healed lepers did), and walk forward, confident in your true identity.

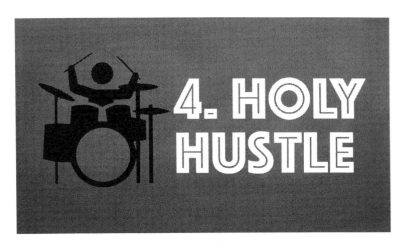

MAIN IDEA= ANY WORK CAN BE SACRED; ANY HUSTLE CAN BE HOLY. WHAT'S THAT MEAN? QUITE SIMPLY, IT'S RESERVED FOR SOMETHING SPECIAL.

GOALS=

- RE-FRAME YOUR WORK AS SACRED. IN WHAT WAYS CAN YOU DO THIS?

- GO "ALL IN" WHEN YOU WORK. WHEN YOU ARE WORKING, DON'T GET DISTRACTED WITH SOCIAL MEDIA, THE TELEVISION, OR ANY OTHER THING.

- WHEN YOU ARE "OFF" GO ALL IN WITH THAT, TOO- NO TEXTING WHILE HANGING OUT WITH THE KIDS, FOR INSTANCE. THIS MAKES ALL AREAS OF LIFE MORE SPECIAL.

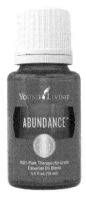

EXPECTATION

APPLY TO WRISTS
OR BACK OF NECK

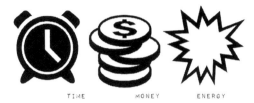

TIME   MONEY   ENERGY

ABUNDANCE

There will never be enough time + money + energy to do everything that COULD be done, but there will always be MORE than enough time + money + energy to do the things that SHOULD be done.

That means you'll not only achieve what you need to achieve, but you'll have margin.

Margin to live unhurried, even as you accomplish your tasks.

Margin to give- and to continue having an abundance.

Margin to mentally process and focus on the things that matter the most.

In other words, you have abundance.

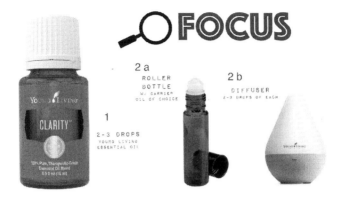

CLARITY

Healthy hustle isn't just knowing when to be off, it's knowing when to be on. Clarity is important.

As you preview your day, apply a few drops of the oil to your wrists and to your neck and/or temples. Inhale the oil on your hands before opening your calendar.

As an option, use in the diffuser (as well).

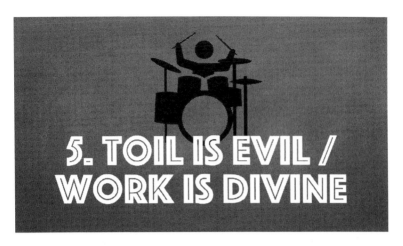

5. TOIL IS EVIL / WORK IS DIVINE

MAIN IDEA= HUSTLE CAN EASILY BECOME TOIL. THE OPPOSITE OF WORK ISN'T LAZINESS. THE OPPOSITE OF WORK IS TOIL. HUSTLE, BUT HUSTLE IN A HEALTHY WAY.

GOALS=

- *DETERMINE NOW WHERE WORK STOPS BECOMING PRODUCTIVE FOR YOU AND WHERE IT BECOMES "TOIL." SET BOUNDARIES.*

- *DECIDE THE THINGS THAT ARE WORTH HUSTLING FOR- AND IDENTIFY THE THINGS THAT ARE NOT. REMEMBER, THERE IS NEVER TIME + ENERGY TO DO EVERYTHING THAT COULD BE DONE, BUT THERE IS ALWAYS MORE THAN ENOUGH TIME + ENERGY TO ACCOMPLISH THE THINGS THAT SHOULD BE DONE.*

- *WHAT DO YOU SEE IN YOUR FUTURE? WHAT ARE YOUR HOPES AND DREAMS?*

- *DO YOU HAVE THE FREEDOM TO DREAM?*

- *AND CAN YOU HUSTLE IN A HEALTHY WAY FOR THOSE DREAMS?*

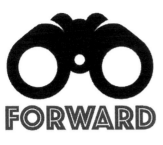

1 3-4 DROPS
ON WRISTS
+ NECK

2 3-4 DROPS
IN DIFFUSER
W/ WATER

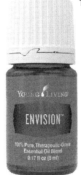

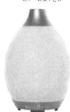

ENVISION

Healthy hustle is about moving forward, about stepping into your destiny. Apply Envision as you begin your work.

Remember why you are hustling…

And remember, when we work in the right way some things get done extremely well, and other things are left undone.

Visioneering empowers us to see the things that need to be done, plan effectively, and then execute strategically to move towards THAT preferred future.

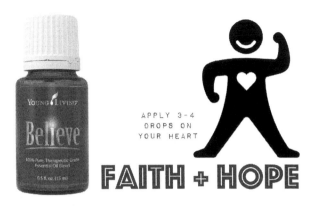

APPLY 3-4
DROPS ON
YOUR HEART

FAITH + HOPE

BELIEVE

Belief can co-exist with doubt. In fact, It almost always does- especially when you're pursuing something grand. You feel like it can happen; you may even know it will happen. But, there's always that smidge of "something else" creeping up.

It helps to remember that your belief isn't just in your ability to get something done. Rather, your belief is placed in the One who works all things together for your good (Romans 8:28), the One- before time began- planned great works for you to walk in (see Ephesians 2:8-10).

NEXT STEPS

Now, you need to acquire the tools to get started. We suggest you order Young Living's Premium Starter Kit (it's an amazing value- it comes with 12 essential oils, a diffuser, and several other items!). You will eventually want the *ten oils for life balance*, too.

If you're able to acquire these at the same time, do so! If not, order the Premium Starter Kit right away- and set an Essential Rewards order for the *oils you'd like to try from this book* to come to you next month. (Essential Rewards is a non-obligation, non-contract program that gives you discounted shipping and points back which you can use for free products. We don't buy anything unless we do it on this program- we love free stuff!).

If you're waiting to purchase the oils, place them on Essential Rewards now and it will ship in approximately 30 days, giving you time to learn the first set of oils. (By placing the order on Essential Rewards, you earn points towards future *free* products!)

To place your order, consult with the person who gave you this material if they are a business-building distributor with Young Living Essential Oils. You will need their coupon code to receive the wholesale discount!

If they are not a distributor OR if you found this info on your own, *please go to* **facebook.com/OilyApp** *and send a PM, or connect through Instagram @OilyApp.*

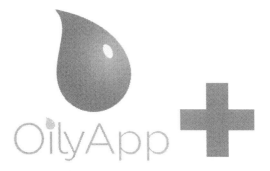

Want to watch the videos that go with this book? And other videos?

OilyApp+ was created for you!

OilyApp+ is a web-based monthly membership / subscription service which provides you with each of the following:

- A monthly class- including a downloadable script AND the videos for the material in this book

- Graphics to match the class!

- 60 second videos to review each of the products mentioned in the class

- Access to Diamond+ leaders and biz-building tips

Here's a deeper dive on each of these features!

CLASSES
= Monthly video + script for you to watch and use on your own!

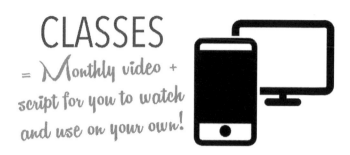

Monthly Feature #1 = An online class you can use to encourage, equip, and empower your team!

Every month- generally, the second week of the month- we go live and teach a class. Here's where it gets good... OilyApp+ subscribers receive forever access to the recording of that class, AS WELL AS the downloadable PDF or script we use.

Join the class simply to learn, or take advantage of the info by passing it on to others!

GRAPHICS
= Our best graphics and copy sent straight to Plus! members

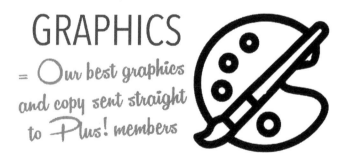

Monthly Feature #2 = Our best graphics available for you to download + share!

We've pulled the best graphics and multi-pic posts from our Instagram feed and placed them where you can download them, then re-use them to share with prospects and grow your business. And, we've included our swipe copy in the files. Use it, edit it, whatever- it's there for you.

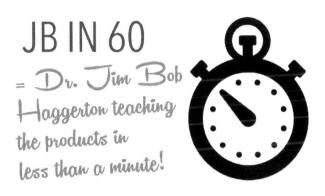

JB IN 60
= Dr. Jim Bob Haggerton teaching the products in less than a minute!

Monthly Feature #3 = How'd you like Dr. Jim Bob Haggerton to teach you about the products?! Done!

Specifically, he'll do it in 60 seconds or less. Whatever products we review in our class- be it the Oils of the Bible, the PSK, the core supplements... he'll give you the 60 second overview of each!

In the online portal, you can login and watch + re-watch as many times as you'd like!

BIZ TIPS

= Videos + more to encourage, equip, and empower you to grow

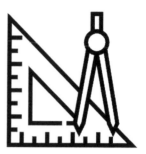

Monthly feature #4 = A recorded video call with one of the top leaders in Young Living! How would you like to hear how one Royal Crown Diamond hit the top rank without ever hosting a class- just by working through social media? Or, how would you like to learn how another did it WITHOUT social media?

What about learning leadership, work-family balance, gaining momentum, or finding your passion form others?

LEADERS

= Exclusive access to top leaders teaching from their wheelhouse!

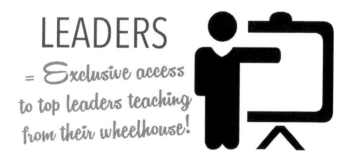

Each month we feature a recorded convo from one of the top leaders teaching from their unique wheelhouse.

Monthly Feature #5 = Bonus videos and other tools we've created to make the biz super-simple and pleasantly practical!

You wouldn't dream of going to work somewhere without understanding how you get paid, and what you can do to make the most of your time. Somehow, we stumble into network marketing and forget to step back and ask those same questions, though.

Each month, we'll drop a resource about the comp plan, about teaching the business, or some other aspect that encourages, equips, and empowers YOU to reach your potential!

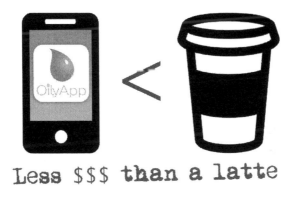

Less $$$ than a latte

You can find all of this on our website- www.OilyApp.com!

And, it's affordable. In fact, it all costs you less than a latte!

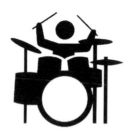

Hustle. Everybody uses the word nowadays, tossing it out like candy on Halloween or cheap beads at Mardi Gras.

But what does it REALLY mean? And how can we ACTUALLY DO IT? And, is there a way to do it and sustain everything else we've got going on in life…?.

Maybe, maybe not. Depends on how you define *hustle.* And it really depends on WHY you're hustling. If you're not careful, it can turn into toil or noise or something worse.

Take the drums in the pic as an example. No musician hustles on stage more than the drummer. They keep the rhythm, they physically push the limits, and they create MUSIC…

But the music happens because of the moments of rest. No rest = all noise.

Rhythm only happens because of the beat of times ON and cadence of times OFF.

Maybe we can learn a lot from the drummer. Maybe we can learn about this thing called hustle and bring some balance in…

In this "short book you'll actually read" we discuss the rhythm of creation (yeah, there really is one), we talk about the wrong reasons we toil, and we determine what healthy hustle looks like. And, in the end, we'll outline ten of the best oils to use for optimal life balance.

Made in the USA
Columbia, SC
25 June 2019